The Handbook for Basic First Aid

Important Note

The information contained within this first aid handbook is intended for informational purposes only and is not intended as a substitute for professional medical advice, diagnosis, or treatment. The author of this handbook and the publisher make no representations or warranties with respect to the accuracy or completeness of the contents of this handbook and specifically disclaim any implied warranties of merchantability or fitness for any particular purpose. The author and publisher shall not be liable for any loss, injury or damage, including, but not limited to, direct, indirect, special, or consequential damages, arising out of, or in any way connected with, the use of the information contained within this handbook. The author and publisher assume no responsibility for any errors or omissions or for any damages resulting from the use of the information contained within this handbook.

This handbook is designed to educate people with basic first aid information, but it is highly recommended that readers take an accredited first aid course to gain a more in-depth understanding of first aid, and emergency medical procedures.

Readers should always consult with a qualified healthcare provider before taking any action based on the information contained within this handbook.

The Importance of Knowing Basic First Aid and Emergency Medicine

Knowing basic first aid and emergency medicine is crucial for anyone, regardless of their profession or position of employment. It is an essential life skill that can save lives and prevent injuries from becoming more serious.

In everyday life, accidents and emergencies can happen unexpectedly and at any time. Knowing basic first aid and emergency medicine can help individuals respond quickly and effectively to these situations. For example, if someone is choking, knowing how to perform the Heimlich maneuver can save their life.

Similarly, if someone is bleeding, knowing how to apply pressure to the wound and elevate the limb can prevent excessive blood loss. Knowing how to recognize signs of a heart attack or stroke and how to perform CPR can help save someone's life until professional medical help arrives.

In a disaster or crisis situation, basic first aid and emergency medicine knowledge can be even more vital. During natural disasters, such as hurricanes, earthquakes, and floods, emergency medical services may not be immediately available. In such situations, knowing basic first aid can help individuals provide medical assistance to themselves and others until help arrives. Knowing how to treat injuries caused by falling debris or how to prevent infection in a contaminated water supply can be crucial in a disaster situation.

Knowing basic first aid and emergency medicine can also help prevent minor injuries from becoming more serious. For example, if someone sprains their ankle, knowing how to properly immobilize the joint and reduce swelling can prevent further damage.

In addition to the personal benefits, knowing basic first aid and emergency medicine can also benefit society as a whole. Don't you want to live in a world where everyone living knew how to save your life in the event you needed saving?

In a community or workplace setting, having individuals trained in basic first aid and emergency medicine can help create a safer environment for everyone. In a school or work setting, having teachers and staff trained in basic first aid can help ensure the safety and well-being of everyone in the school or workplace.

Knowing basic first aid and emergency medicine is an essential life skill that can save lives and provide peace of mind in an emergency situation. It is vital for individuals to take the time to learn basic first aid and emergency medicine if we want to create a safer world for everyone who stands to inherit it after us.

The Difference Between First Aid and Emergency Medicine

First aid is a set of emergency procedures that are performed in order to provide immediate medical assistance to someone who is injured or ill. It is the initial response to an injury or illness and is designed to preserve life, prevent further injury or illness, and promote recovery. First aid can include a wide range of procedures, from basic life support (such as CPR) to treating minor injuries (such as cuts and bruises).

Emergency medicine, on the other hand, is a branch of medicine that is focused on providing immediate medical care to individuals in critical or emergency situations. Emergency medicine physicians and nurses are trained to quickly assess, diagnose, and treat patients who have urgent medical needs. They are often the first medical professionals on the scene in emergency situations, such as car accidents, natural disasters, and heart attacks. Emergency medicine professionals are also responsible for stabilizing patients and preparing them for transport to a hospital or other medical facility.

While first aid and emergency medicine are related, they are not the same thing. First aid is the initial response to an injury or illness, while emergency medicine is the specialized care that is provided by trained medical professionals. First aid can be performed by anyone, whereas emergency medicine is typically performed by trained medical professionals such as paramedics, nurses, and doctors.

In summary, first aid is the immediate and temporary care given to someone who is injured or ill before professional medical help arrives. Emergency medicine is the specialized care provided by trained medical professionals to individuals in critical or emergency situations. Both first aid and emergency medicine are important to preserve life, prevent further injury or illness, and promote recovery.

Basic First Aid

There are many types of basic first aid, but some common types include:

Cardiopulmonary Resuscitation (CPR): This involves chest compressions and rescue breathing to help circulate oxygen to the brain and keep the heart beating in case of cardiac arrest.

Choking: This involves performing the Heimlich maneuver to dislodge an object blocking the airway.

Bleeding: This involves applying pressure to the wound and elevating the limb to stop blood loss.

Burns: This involves cooling the burn with water, covering it with a sterile dressing, and elevating the affected limb if it is a limb burn.

Fractures: This involves immobilizing the affected limb using a splint or sling to prevent further injury.

Head injuries: This involves keeping the person still, monitoring their condition and vital signs and seeking medical attention if necessary.

Shock: This involves elevating the person's feet, keeping them warm, and seeking medical attention if necessary.

Sprains and strains: This involves rest, ice, compression, and elevation of the affected limb.

Poisoning: This involves identifying the source of the poison, calling for medical help and providing supportive care until professional help arrives.

Heat stroke: This involves moving the person to a cool place, removing any unnecessary clothing, providing them with water or sports drinks and seeking medical attention if necessary.

Hypothermia: This involves moving the person to a warm place, removing any wet clothing, providing them with warm beverages and seeking medical attention if necessary.

Seizures: This involves keeping the person safe by removing any nearby objects, protecting their head, and timing the seizure.

Insect bites and stings: The treatment for insect bites and stings depends on the type of insect, the severity of the bite or sting, and the person's individual reaction.

Anaphylaxis: Anaphylaxis is a severe and potentially life-threatening allergic reaction characterized by symptoms such as difficulty breathing, hives, swelling of the face, lips, or throat, and in some cases, a sudden drop in blood pressure and loss of consciousness.

Diabetic Emergency: A diabetes emergency is a life-threatening condition caused by either high or low blood sugar levels and characterized by symptoms such as confusion, unconsciousness, seizures and difficulty breathing.

Cardiopulmonary Resuscitation (CPR)

Cardiopulmonary Resuscitation (CPR) is a life-saving procedure that can be performed by anyone. It is used to restore blood flow and breathing in someone whose heart has stopped beating (cardiac arrest). The goal of CPR is to keep oxygenated blood flowing to the brain and other vital organs until professional medical help arrives.

Here are the steps to perform CPR:

Determine unresponsiveness: Check to see if the person is responsive by tapping their shoulder and speaking loudly to them. If they do not respond, they may be in cardiac arrest.

Call for emergency medical services:
Call 911 or your local emergency number immediately. If someone else is present, have them call for help while you begin CPR.

Check for breathing: Look, listen, and feel for breathing by placing your ear near the person's nose and mouth and looking at their chest to see if it is rising and falling. If the person is not breathing, begin CPR.

Begin chest compressions: Position yourself with your hands on the person's chest. Place the heel of one hand on the center of the person's chest, and the heel of your other hand on top of the first hand. Interlock your fingers and keep your elbows straight. Press down on the chest with your body weight to compress the chest about 2 inches. Release the pressure, and let the chest rise to its normal position. Repeat these compressions at a rate of about 100-120 compressions per minute.

Provide rescue breathing: After 30 compressions, open the person's airway by tilting their head back and lifting their chin. Pinch the person's nose closed, and take a deep breath. Seal your lips around their mouth and blow into their lungs until you see their chest rise. Give two breaths, then continue with 30 more compressions.

Continue CPR: Continue performing chest compressions and rescue breathing in cycles of 30 compressions and 2 breaths until professional help arrives or the person begins to breathe on their own.

It's important to note that performing CPR can be tiring, and if you are performing it alone, it's important to take breaks or rotate with another person if possible. Also, if you are not trained in CPR, it's important to know that chest compressions alone can also help save a life and it's better to perform them than to do nothing.

CPR can be the difference between life and death in a cardiac arrest situation, and it's important for everyone to know how to perform it. It's also important to note that CPR guidelines change over time, and it's good to refresh your knowledge and skills by taking a CPR course regularly.

Choking

Choking occurs when an object becomes lodged in the airway, preventing air from flowing into the lungs. It is a serious medical emergency that requires immediate attention. Here are the steps to perform first aid for someone choking:

Determine if the person is choking: Look for the universal choking sign, which is the person holding their throat with one or both hands and making loud coughing sounds or gagging.

Encourage the person to cough: If the person is able to cough, encourage them to continue coughing. Coughing can help dislodge the object from the airway.

Perform the Heimlich maneuver: If the person is unable to cough or speak, or if their coughing becomes ineffective, you should perform the Heimlich maneuver. To perform the Heimlich maneuver:

- Stand behind the person and wrap your arms around their waist.
- Make a fist with one hand and place it just above the person's navel.
- Grasp your fist with your other hand.
- Press your fist into the person's abdomen with a sudden upward thrust.
- Repeat the thrusts until the object is dislodged or the person starts to breathe.

Check the airway: After the object is dislodged, check the person's airway to make sure it is clear. If the person is still not breathing, begin CPR.

Seek medical attention: Even if the person starts breathing again, it is important to seek medical attention. The object may have caused damage to the airway, and the person may require further medical treatment.

It's important to note that it is better to perform the Heimlich maneuver than to do nothing, if the person is choking and unable to cough or speak, even if you are not sure if the Heimlich maneuver is needed. Also, if you are alone and choking, it's possible to perform the Heimlich maneuver on yourself by using a solid object such as a chair or countertop to push against your abdomen.

Knowing how to perform the Heimlich maneuver can be the difference between life and death in a choking emergency, and it's important for everyone to know how to perform it. It's also important to note that choking guidelines change over time, and it's good to refresh your knowledge and skills by taking a first aid course regularly.

Bleeding

Bleeding occurs when a blood vessel is damaged, causing blood to flow out of the body. It can be caused by a variety of factors, including cuts, scrapes, puncture wounds, and fractures. If not treated properly, bleeding can lead to serious complications such as shock and organ failure. Here are the steps to perform first aid for someone bleeding:

Assess the situation: Make sure that you and the person are safe. If the person is in a dangerous situation, try to move them to a safe location.

Identify the source of the bleeding: Look for the source of the bleeding, such as a cut or puncture wound.

Apply direct pressure: Apply direct pressure to the wound with a clean cloth, tissue or gauze. Use your hand to press down on the wound firmly to help stop the bleeding.

Elevate the limb: If the wound is on an arm or leg, elevate the limb above the level of the person's heart to help reduce blood flow to the wound.

Apply a pressure bandage: Once the bleeding has stopped or slowed, apply a pressure bandage.

Apply a tourniquet: If the bleeding is severe, and direct pressure and elevation are not stopping the bleeding, you can use a tourniquet. A tourniquet is a device that is used to stop the flow of blood through an artery. A tourniquet should only be used as a last resort, as it can cause damage to the limb if left on for too long.

Monitor the person's vital signs: While providing first aid, keep monitoring the person's vital signs such as pulse, breathing and consciousness level.

Seek medical attention: Even if the bleeding has stopped or slowed, it is important to seek medical attention. The wound may require further treatment to prevent infection and promote healing.

It's important to note that if the bleeding is caused by a puncture wound, it is important not to remove the object that caused the wound, if it is still in place. Doing so can cause more bleeding and damage. Instead, apply pressure around the object.

Bleeding can be a serious emergency, and prompt first aid is essential to prevent excessive blood loss and to preserve life.

Burns

Burns are a common injury that can be caused by heat, chemicals, electricity, or radiation. They can range from minor to severe, and the severity of the burn will determine the appropriate first aid treatment. Here are the steps to perform first aid for someone who has suffered a burn:

Assess the situation: Make sure that you and the person are safe. If the person is in a dangerous situation, try to move them to a safe location.

Identify the type of burn: Burns can be classified as first-degree, second-degree, or third-degree:

- First-degree burns are characterized by redness, mild pain, and no blistering. They are usually minor and can be treated at home.

- Second-degree burns are characterized by redness, pain, and blistering. They are deeper than first-degree burns and require medical attention.

- Third-degree burns are characterized by white or blackened skin, no pain, and no sensation. They are the most severe type of burn and require immediate medical attention.

Stop the burning: If the person's clothing is on fire, have them stop, drop, and roll to extinguish the flames. If the burn was caused by a hot liquid or steam, remove the person from the source of the heat.

Cool the burn: Cool the burn by running cool water over it for at least 20 minutes. This helps to reduce pain and inflammation, and prevent further tissue damage.

Cover the burn: Once the burn has been cooled, cover it with a sterile, non-adhesive dressing.

Monitor the person's vital signs: Keep monitoring the person's vital signs such as pulse breathing and consciousness level.

Seek medical attention: If the burn is severe, or covers a large area of the body, or on the face, hands, feet or genitals, seek medical attention immediately.

It's important to note that you should never use ice, butter or ointment to cool a burn, as they can cause further damage to the skin. Also, avoid breaking any blisters that form on the burn, as they help to protect the wound from infection. Burns can be a serious injury, and prompt first aid is essential to prevent infection and to promote healing.

Fractures

A bone fracture is a break or crack in a bone. It can occur as a result of a fall, a blow to the bone, or overuse. The appropriate first aid treatment for a bone fracture will depend on the location and severity of the fracture. Here are the steps to perform first aid for someone who has suffered a bone fracture:

Assess the situation: Make sure that you and the person are safe. If the person is in a dangerous situation, try to move them to a safe location.

Identify the location of the fracture: Look for signs of a fracture such as deformity, swelling, or pain at the site of the injury.

Immobilize the fracture: Immobilize the fracture by splinting or using a sling to keep the bone in place. You can use anything that is firm and straight, such as a stick, a rolled-up magazine, or a piece of cardboard.

Apply ice: Apply ice to the area to reduce swelling and pain. Wrap the ice in a towel or cloth and place it on the area for 15-20 minutes at a time.

Monitor vital signs: Keep monitoring the person's vital signs such as pulse, breathing and consciousness level.

Seek medical attention: Even if the fracture appears to be minor, it is important to seek medical attention. A healthcare professional can properly examine the fracture and provide appropriate treatment.

It's important to note that if the bone is protruding through the skin, or if the limb looks deformed, or if the person is experiencing numbness or tingling, do not attempt to move the limb or realign the bone. Instead, keep the person still and immobilize the limb as best as you can.

A bone fracture can be a serious injury, and prompt first aid is essential to prevent further injury, to reduce pain and to promote healing.

Head Injuries

A head injury is an injury to the head or brain that can occur as a result of a fall, a blow to the head, or a car accident. The appropriate first aid treatment for a head injury will depend on the severity of the injury. Here are the steps to perform first aid for someone who has suffered a head injury:

Assess the situation: Make sure that you and the person are safe. If the person is in a dangerous situation, try to move them to a safe location.

Check for consciousness: Tap the person's shoulder and speak to them in a loud voice. If the person does not respond, they may be unconscious.

Call for emergency medical services: Call 911 or your local emergency number immediately. If someone else is present, have them call for help while you begin first aid.

Keep the person still: Keep the person still and do not move them unless it is absolutely necessary. Moving a person with a head injury can cause further damage.

Check for breathing: Look, listen, and feel for breathing by placing your ear near the person's nose and mouth and looking at their chest to see if it is rising and falling. If the person is not breathing, begin CPR.

Monitor vital signs: Keep monitoring the person's vital signs such as pulse, breathing and consciousness level.

Seek medical attention: Even if the person appears to be fine, it is important to seek medical attention. A healthcare professional can properly examine the person and provide appropriate treatment.

It's important to note that a person with a head injury may not show symptoms immediately, and some symptoms may appear hours or days after the injury. Therefore, it's important to keep an eye on the person and to seek medical attention if symptoms such as headache, nausea, confusion, or loss of consciousness appear.

A head injury can be a serious injury, and prompt first aid is essential to prevent further damage to the brain, to reduce pain and to promote healing. It's important for anyone who may be in a situation where a head injury could occur, such as sports or any physical activity, to know how to perform basic first aid for head injuries and to refresh their knowledge and skills by taking a first aid course regularly.

Shock

Shock is a medical emergency that occurs when the body is not getting enough blood flow. This can happen due to a variety of reasons such as injury, bleeding, infection, or severe allergic reactions. The person may appear pale, have cold and clammy skin, rapid heartbeat, low blood pressure, confusion, and difficulty breathing. Here are the steps to perform first aid for someone who is suffering from shock:

Assess the situation: Make sure that you and the person are safe. If the person is in a dangerous situation, try to move them to a safe location.

Call for emergency medical services: Call 911 or your local emergency number immediately. If someone else is present, have them call for help while you begin first aid.

Keep the person still: Keep the person still and do not move them unless it is absolutely necessary. Moving a person in shock can cause further damage.

Elevate the person's legs: If the person is lying down, raise their legs about 12 inches to help improve blood flow to the brain.

Keep the person warm: Keep the person warm by covering them with a blanket or other warm covering.

Monitor vital signs: Keep monitoring the person's vital signs such as pulse, breathing and consciousness level.

Seek medical attention: Even if the person appears to be fine, it is important to seek medical attention. A healthcare professional can properly examine the person and provide appropriate treatment.

It's important to note that the person in shock should be transported to the hospital as soon as possible for further treatment. While waiting for emergency services to arrive, it's important to keep the person still, keep them warm, and monitor their vital signs. Also, if the person is conscious, it's important to provide them with reassurance and support.

Shock can be caused by a variety of underlying conditions, so it's important for emergency medical services to determine the cause and provide the appropriate treatment. It's also important to know that shock can be life-threatening if not treated promptly, and the first aid measures mentioned above are just temporary measures until professional medical help arrives.

Sprains and Strains

A sprain occurs when the ligaments that connect bones are stretched or torn, while a strain is an injury to a muscle or tendon. Sprains and strains can occur as a result of a fall, a twist, or overuse. The appropriate first aid treatment for a sprain or strain will depend on the severity of the injury. Here are the steps to perform first aid for someone who has suffered a sprain or strain:

Assess the situation: Make sure that you and the person are safe. If the person is in a dangerous situation, try to move them to a safe location.

Identify the location of the injury: Look for signs of a sprain or strain such as pain, swelling, or bruising.

Rest the affected area: Rest the affected area and avoid any activity that causes pain.

Ice the area: Apply ice to the area to reduce swelling and pain. Wrap the ice in a towel or cloth and place it on the area for 15-20 minutes at a time.

Compress the area: Use a bandage or an elastic bandage to compress the area and help reduce swelling.

Elevate the area: If the injury is to a limb, elevate the limb above the level of the person's heart to help reduce blood flow to the area.

Monitor vital signs: Keep monitoring the person's vital signs such as pulse, breathing and consciousness level.

Seek medical attention: Even if the injury appears to be minor, it is important to seek medical attention. A healthcare professional can properly examine the injury and provide appropriate treatment.

It's important to note that while waiting for medical attention, it's important to avoid any activities that cause pain, and to keep the affected area immobilized. Also, if the pain, swelling or bruising is severe or if the person is unable to move the affected area, it's recommended to seek medical attention immediately. A sprain or strain can be a painful injury, and prompt first aid is essential to prevent further injury, to reduce pain and to promote healing.

Poisoning

Poisoning occurs when a person ingests, inhales, or comes into contact with a substance that is harmful to their body. The appropriate first aid treatment for poisoning will depend on the type of poison and the severity of the poisoning. Here are the steps to perform first aid for someone who has suffered from poisoning:

Assess the situation: Make sure that you and the person are safe. If the person is in a dangerous situation, try to move them to a safe location.

Call for emergency medical services: Call 911 or your local emergency number immediately. If someone else is present, have them call for help while you begin first aid.

Identify the poison: If possible, try to identify the poison by looking at the packaging or by asking the person.

Keep the person still: Keep the person still and do not move them unless it is absolutely necessary. Moving a person in shock can cause further damage.

Remove the poison: If the poison is on the skin or in the eyes, remove any clothing that may be contaminated and flush the skin or eyes with water for at least 20 minutes. If the person has ingested the poison, do not induce vomiting unless instructed to do so by a healthcare professional.

Monitor vital signs: Keep monitoring the person's vital signs such as pulse, breathing and consciousness level.

Seek medical attention: Even if the person appears to be fine, it is important to seek medical attention. A healthcare professional can properly examine the person and provide appropriate treatment.

It's important to note that if the person is unconscious, not breathing, or having seizures, provide CPR if you are trained. Also, it's important to bring the poison container or a sample of the poison, if possible, to the emergency room for identification and proper treatment.

Heat Stroke

Heat stroke occurs when the body is unable to regulate its temperature due to prolonged exposure to high temperatures. It can be a life-threatening condition, and prompt first aid is essential to prevent further damage to the body. Here are the steps to perform first aid for someone who is suffering from heat stroke:

Assess the situation: Make sure that you and the person are safe. If the person is in a dangerous situation, try to move them to a safe location.

Call for emergency medical services: Call 911 or your local emergency number immediately. If someone else is present, have them call for help while you begin first aid.

Move the person to a cool place: Move the person to a shaded or air-conditioned area, or place them in front of a fan.

Remove excess clothing: Remove any excess clothing to help cool the person's body.

Apply cool water: Apply cool water to the person's skin, such as by using a damp cloth or by spraying them with a water bottle.

Monitor vital signs: Keep monitoring the person's vital signs such as pulse, breathing and consciousness level.

Seek medical attention: Even if the person appears to be fine, it is important to seek medical attention. A healthcare professional can properly examine the person and provide appropriate treatment.

It's important to note that if the person is unconscious, not breathing, or having seizures, provide CPR if you are trained. Also, if the person's temperature rises above 104 degrees Fahrenheit, it's important to seek medical attention immediately.

Heat stroke can be a serious condition and can be caused by various factors such as high temperatures, dehydration, and certain medications. The symptoms of heat stroke include high body temperature, hot and dry skin, dizziness, nausea, confusion, and unconsciousness. It's important for everyone to know how to recognize the signs of heat stroke and to perform basic first aid to prevent further damage to the body.

Heat exhaustion is a condition that occurs when the body is unable to regulate its temperature due to prolonged exposure to high temperatures. It is characterized by symptoms such as heavy sweating, weakness, dizziness, nausea, headache, and muscle cramps. It's a less severe form of heat-related illness than heat stroke, but it still requires prompt treatment. Follow the first aid for someone who is suffering from heat exhaustion as mentioned above, and for both situations, provide fluids. Offer the person fluids such as water or an electrolyte-replacement drink, to help rehydrate them and replace any fluids lost through sweating.

Hypothermia

Hypothermia is a condition that occurs when the body's temperature drops below normal, often caused by prolonged exposure to cold temperatures. It can be a life-threatening condition, and prompt first aid is essential to prevent further damage to the body. Here are the steps to perform first aid for someone who is suffering from hypothermia:

Assess the situation: Make sure that you and the person are safe. If the person is in a dangerous situation, try to move them to a safe location.

Call for emergency medical services: Call 911 or your local emergency number immediately. If someone else is present, have them call for help while you begin first aid.

Move the person to a warm place: Move the person to a warm, dry place, such as a warm room or vehicle.

Remove any wet clothing: Remove any wet clothing and replace it with warm, dry clothing or a blanket.

Provide warmth: Use a blanket or other warm covering to keep the person warm. You can also use a hot water bottle or a heating pad, placed on the person's chest, neck, or groin area, to help raise the person's core temperature.

Provide fluids: Offer the person warm fluids such as water or broth, if they are conscious and able to swallow.

Monitor vital signs: Keep monitoring the person's vital signs such as pulse, breathing and consciousness level.

Seek medical attention: Even if the person appears to be fine, it is important to seek medical attention. A healthcare professional can properly examine the person and provide appropriate treatment.

It's important to note that if the person is unconscious, not breathing, or having seizures, provide CPR if you are trained. Also, if the person's temperature is below 95 degrees Fahrenheit (35 degrees Celsius), it's important to seek medical attention immediately.

Hypothermia can be caused by various factors such as cold temperatures, wet clothing, and certain medical conditions. It's important for everyone to know how to recognize the signs of hypothermia and to

perform basic first aid to prevent further
damage to the body.

Seizures

A seizure is a sudden, uncontrolled electrical disturbance in the brain that can cause a variety of symptoms such as convulsions, muscle contractions, loss of consciousness, and changes in behavior. Seizures can be caused by a variety of factors such as epilepsy, head injury, stroke, fever, or certain medical conditions. The appropriate first aid treatment for a seizure will depend on the cause of the seizure and the severity of the symptoms. Here are the steps to perform first aid for someone who is suffering from a seizure:

Assess the situation: Make sure that you and the person are safe. If the person is in a dangerous situation, try to move them to a safe location.

Clear the area around the person: Clear the area around the person of any sharp or hard objects, to prevent injury.

Do not restrain the person: Do not try to restrain the person during a seizure, as this can cause injury.

Protect the person's head: Use a pillow or a piece of clothing to protect the person's head from injury.

Time the seizure: Time the seizure, as seizures usually last a few minutes.

Monitor vital signs: Keep monitoring the person's vital signs such as pulse, breathing and consciousness level.

Seek medical attention: Even if the seizure appears to be minor, it is important to seek medical attention. A healthcare professional can properly examine the person and provide appropriate treatment.

It's important to note that if the person is unconscious, not breathing, or having seizures lasting longer than 5 minutes, call for emergency medical services immediately. Also, if the person is prone to seizures, it's important to inform the emergency services about it and if the person has a medical ID or a seizure action plan.

Insect Bites and Stings

Insect bites and stings can cause a variety of symptoms such as pain, itching, swelling, and redness. They can also cause more serious reactions such as an allergic reaction. The appropriate first aid treatment for insect bites and stings will depend on the severity of the symptoms. Here are the steps to perform first aid for someone who is suffering from insect bites and stings:

Clean the area: Use soap and water to clean the area around the bite or sting. This can help prevent infection.

Remove the stinger: If the insect has left a stinger, remove it as soon as possible.

This can help reduce the amount of venom that enters the skin.

Clean the area: Clean the area of the bite or sting with soap and water.

Apply a cold compress: Applying a cold compress (such as a bag of ice or a cold pack) to the area can help reduce pain and swelling.

Use over-the-counter medication: Over-the-counter medications such as ibuprofen or acetaminophen can help reduce pain and inflammation.

Apply a cream or lotion: Some creams and lotions can be applied to the area to help reduce itching and inflammation.

Watch for signs of an allergic reaction: If the person experience severe symptoms such as difficulty breathing, hives, or swelling of the face or throat, they should seek medical attention immediately.

Keep an eye on the bite or sting: Keep an eye on the bite or sting for the next 24 to 48 hours to make sure that it does not become infected or cause other symptoms.

It's important to note that some people may have a severe allergic reaction to insect bites and stings, which is called anaphylaxis, and they should carry an epinephrine auto-injector (EpiPen) with them and know how to use it in case of an emergency.

Anaphylaxis

Anaphylaxis is a severe and potentially life-threatening allergic reaction. If someone witnesses someone suffering from anaphylaxis, they should take immediate action to provide first aid and call for emergency medical assistance. Here are the steps to perform first aid for someone who is suffering from anaphylaxis:

Call for emergency medical services: Dial 911 or your local emergency number immediately. If someone else is present, have them call for help while you begin first aid.

Administer epinephrine: If the person has an EpiPen, or another form of injectable epinephrine, help them use it as soon as possible. Epinephrine is the first-line treatment for anaphylaxis and can help to reduce the severity of the reaction.

Help the person sit or lie down: Help the person to sit or lie down in a comfortable position, with their legs elevated if possible. This can help to improve blood flow and reduce the risk of shock.

Loosen any tight clothing: Help the person to loosen any tight clothing, such as a belt or a collar, to help them breathe more easily.

Monitor vital signs: Keep monitoring the person's vital signs such as pulse, breathing and consciousness level.

Stay with the person: Stay with the person until emergency medical services arrive. Keep them calm and reassure them that help is on the way.

Follow up with medical attention: Even if the person appears to be fine, it is important to seek medical attention after an anaphylactic episode. A healthcare professional can properly examine the person and provide appropriate treatment.

It's important to note that if the person is unconscious, not breathing, or having seizures, provide CPR if you are trained. Also, anaphylaxis can be caused by various allergens such as food, medications, insect stings, and certain medical conditions. The symptoms of anaphylaxis include difficulty breathing, hives, swelling of the face, lips, or throat, and in some cases, it can cause a sudden drop in blood pressure and loss of consciousness.

Diabetic Emergency

A diabetes emergency can be caused by a variety of factors such as high or low blood sugar levels, and it can be a life-threatening condition. If someone witnesses someone suffering from a diabetes emergency, they should take immediate action to provide first aid and call for emergency medical assistance. Here are the steps to perform first aid for someone who is suffering from a diabetes emergency:

Call for emergency medical services: Dial 911 or your local emergency number immediately. If someone else is present, have them call for help while you begin first aid.

Identify the type of emergency: If the person is conscious, ask them about their symptoms and try to identify if the emergency is related to high blood sugar (hyperglycemia) or low blood sugar (hypoglycemia).

Treat hypoglycemia: If the person is suffering from hypoglycemia (low blood sugar), give them a fast-acting source of sugar such as glucose tablets, fruit juice, or regular soda. If the person is unconscious, do not give them anything to eat or drink.

Treat hyperglycemia: If the person is suffering from hyperglycemia (high blood sugar), give them insulin as prescribed by their healthcare provider and help them to monitor their blood sugar levels.

Monitor vital signs: Keep monitoring the person's vital signs such as pulse, breathing and consciousness level.

Stay with the person: Stay with the person until emergency medical services arrive. Keep them calm and reassure them that help is on the way.

Follow up with medical attention: Even if the person appears to be fine, it is important to seek medical attention after a diabetes emergency. A healthcare professional can properly examine the person and provide appropriate treatment.

It's important to note that if the person is unconscious, not breathing, or having seizures, provide CPR if you are trained. Also, if the person has a medical ID or a diabetes action plan, inform the emergency services about it.

Common Illnesses

Cold, flu, and fever are common illnesses that can cause a variety of symptoms such as a runny nose, cough, sore throat, fever, and fatigue. The appropriate first aid treatment for these illnesses will depend on the severity of the symptoms. Here are the steps to perform first aid for someone who is suffering from a cold, flu, or fever:

Encourage rest: Help the person to get plenty of rest. This can help to speed up recovery and reduce the risk of complications.

Provide fluids: Help the person to stay hydrated by providing fluids such as water, juice, and clear broths. This can help to prevent dehydration and soothe a sore throat.

Use over-the-counter medication: Give the person over-the-counter medication such as acetaminophen or ibuprofen to reduce fever and relieve pain.

Use a humidifier: Use a humidifier to add moisture to the air, which can help to ease congestion and soothe a sore throat.

Keep the person comfortable: Keep the person comfortable by providing a warm blanket, and keeping the room at a comfortable temperature.

Monitor vital signs: Keep monitoring the person's vital signs such as temperature, pulse, and breathing.

Seek medical attention: If the person's symptoms worsen or if they are at risk of complications, seek medical attention.

Prevent the spread of infection: To prevent the spread of infection, make sure the person covers their mouth and nose when they cough or sneeze, and wash their hands frequently.

It's important to note that if the person is having difficulty breathing, chest pain or pressure, severe headache, neck stiffness or a rash, or is confused, or unconscious, call for emergency medical services immediately.

It's also important for people to practice good hygiene, get enough rest and stay healthy by eating a balanced diet and getting regular exercise.

When to Seek Medical Help

It is important to seek medical help when a person is experiencing symptoms that are severe, persistent, or unusual, or when a person's condition worsens or does not improve with self-care or over-the-counter medication. It is also important to seek medical help if the person has a pre-existing medical condition, is pregnant, elderly, or has a weakened immune system.

Here are some signs that a situation is serious and requires professional medical attention:

- Difficulty breathing, chest pain or pressure

- Severe headache, neck stiffness, or a rash
- Confusion, or unconsciousness
- Severe abdominal pain, vomiting, or diarrhea
- Sudden or severe pain, swelling, or bleeding
- High fever, or fever that lasts for more than a few days
- Persistent or severe coughing, chest congestion, or difficulty breathing
- Persistent or severe vomiting, or difficulty keeping fluids down
- Persistent or severe diarrhea, or blood in the stool
- Sudden or severe allergic reactions
- Signs of infection such as redness, swelling, warmth, or pus
- Persistent or severe fatigue, weakness, or dizziness

- Persistent or severe anxiety, depression, or other emotional distress

It's important to note that if the person is having difficulty breathing, chest pain or pressure, severe headache, neck stiffness or a rash, or is confused, or unconscious, call for emergency medical services immediately. It's also important to know when a situation is serious and requires professional medical attention as this can prevent further damage to the body and help to ensure a timely and effective treatment.

Tips for Preventing Common Illnesses and Injuries

Here are some tips for preventing common illnesses and injuries:

Wash your hands regularly: Washing your hands with soap and water is one of the most effective ways to prevent the spread of germs and infections.

Practice good hygiene: Practice good hygiene habits such as keeping your hands away from your face, avoiding close contact with people who are sick, and covering your mouth and nose when you cough or sneeze.

Get enough sleep: Getting enough sleep is important for maintaining a healthy immune system and reducing the risk of illnesses and injuries.

Exercise regularly: Regular exercise can help to boost your immune system, improve your overall health, and reduce the risk of injuries.

Eat a balanced diet: Eating a balanced diet that is rich in fruits, vegetables, and whole grains can help to maintain a healthy immune system and reduce the risk of illnesses and injuries.

Avoid smoking and excessive alcohol consumption: Smoking and excessive alcohol consumption can increase the risk of illnesses and injuries.

Get vaccinated: Getting vaccinated can help to protect you from a variety of serious and sometimes life-threatening illnesses.

Keep a first-aid kit: Keep a first-aid kit at home and know how to use it in case of an emergency.

Wear appropriate safety gear: When engaging in activities such as sports or cycling, wear the appropriate safety gear to reduce the risk of injuries.

Be aware of your surroundings: Be aware of your surroundings and take steps to reduce the risk of accidents and injuries, such as keeping walkways clear of obstacles and properly maintaining equipment.

It's also important to recognize the early signs of illnesses and injuries and to seek medical attention when necessary. By following these tips, you can reduce your risk of common illnesses and injuries, and improve your overall health and well-being.

How to Prepare for an Emergency

Preparing for emergencies can help to ensure that you are able to respond quickly and effectively in the event of an emergency. Here are some steps to take to prepare for emergencies:

Create an emergency plan: Develop an emergency plan with your family that includes a designated meeting place, emergency contact information, and evacuation routes.

Assemble an emergency kit: Assemble an emergency kit that includes items such as food, water, first-aid supplies, a flashlight, and a battery-powered radio.

Stay informed: Stay informed about potential emergencies by listening to local news and weather reports, and signing up for local alerts and notifications.

Learn first aid and CPR: Learn first aid and CPR so that you can provide immediate medical assistance in case of an emergency.

Identify emergency services: Identify the emergency services in your area, such as the police, fire department, and local hospital, and make sure you know the phone number for emergency services.

Familiarize yourself with emergency evacuation routes: Familiarize yourself with emergency evacuation routes and make sure you know how to get to safety in case of an emergency.

Keep important documents in a safe place: Keep important documents such as identification, insurance policies, and emergency contact information in a safe place where they can be easily accessed in case of an emergency.

Practice your emergency plan: Regularly practice your emergency plan so that you and your family are prepared to respond quickly and effectively in case of an emergency.

Have a communication plan: Have a communication plan in case of emergency, so that you can check on your loved ones and let them know you are safe.

By taking these steps, you can be better prepared for emergencies and increase your chances of staying safe in the event of an emergency. It's also important to be aware of the potential emergencies that might happen in your area, such as natural disasters, power outages, and regularly update your emergency plan and emergency kit.

Basic First Aid Supply List

Here is a basic first aid supplies list that can be used as a guide to assemble a first aid kit:

Adhesive bandages: Various sizes of adhesive bandages to cover cuts and scrapes.

Antiseptic wipes: To clean wounds and prevent infection.

Antibiotic ointment: To prevent infection in minor cuts, scrapes, and burns.

Tweezers: To remove splinters and other foreign objects from the skin.

Scissors: To cut gauze, tape, and clothing.

Disposable gloves: To protect yourself and others from blood-borne pathogens.

CPR face shield: To protect yourself while performing CPR.

Instant cold pack: To reduce swelling and pain from sprains and strains.

Digital thermometer: To measure body temperature.

Pain relievers: such as ibuprofen or acetaminophen for minor aches and pain

Elastic bandage: To provide support and compression to sprains and strains

Sterile gauze pads and adhesive tape: To cover and protect wounds.

Splint: To immobilize fractures and dislocations

Flashlight: To provide light in case of power outages or low visibility.

Emergency blanket: To keep the person warm

This list is a guide and it may vary depending on the location and the type of activities that you are doing. It's important to keep the first aid kit in a convenient place, such as a backpack, purse or car, and to regularly check the contents and replace any expired or missing items. It's also important to take a first aid course to learn how to properly use the items in the kit and how to respond in case of an emergency.

Common Medications and Their Uses

Here is a list of common medications and their uses:

Acetaminophen (Tylenol): Used to relieve pain and reduce fever.

Ibuprofen (Advil, Motrin): Used to relieve pain, reduce fever, and reduce inflammation.

Aspirin: Used to relieve pain, reduce fever, and reduce inflammation. It also used as a blood thinner.

Diphenhydramine (Benadryl): Used to relieve symptoms of allergies, such as sneezing, runny nose, and itchy eyes. It's also used as a sleep aid.

Loratadine (Claritin): Used to relieve symptoms of allergies, such as sneezing, runny nose, and itchy eyes.

Pseudoephedrine (Sudafed): Used to relieve nasal congestion caused by colds, flu, and allergies.

Dextromethorphan (Robitussin): Used to relieve coughing.

Cetirizine (Zyrtec): Used to relieve symptoms of allergies, such as sneezing, runny nose, and itchy eyes.

Albuterol (ProAir, Ventolin): Used to open up the airways in the lungs to make breathing easier for people with asthma and other lung diseases.

Diphenoxylate (Lomotil): Used to treat diarrhea.

Metformin (Glucophage): Used to treat type 2 diabetes.

Insulin: Used to treat type 1 diabetes, and some type 2 diabetes.

Amoxicillin: An antibiotic used to treat bacterial infections

Prednisone: A steroid used to reduce inflammation and treat various conditions such as asthma, allergies and some types of cancer.

Omeprazole (Prilosec): A medication used to reduce stomach acid and treat conditions such as acid reflux and ulcers.

It's important to note that this list is not exhaustive and that medications should only be taken under the guidance of a healthcare professional. Additionally, it's important to read the label and follow the instructions carefully, and to inform your healthcare professional of any other

medications or supplements you are
taking.

Alternative Medicines

There are many alternative medicines that require extensive knowledge in order to practice them safely and effectively. So much knowledge, that an entire additional book is required to explain it. With that being said, imagine you were stranded in the deep bush for sixty days. It would be helpful to know what surrounding plants could provide you with the resources you needed in the moment, without access to any pharmaceutical medications.

Considering this hypothetical, it is still very important to remember that this is just a list of useful plants. It is not a replacement for first aid. Extra study is required to effectively implement and use these plants safe and effectively:

Aloe vera: Used for treating burns, skin irritations, and cuts.

Calendula: Used for treating skin irritations, cuts, and bruises.

Echinacea: Used for boosting the immune system and fighting infections.

Garlic: Used for its antibacterial and antiviral properties.

Ginger: Used for treating digestive problems and nausea.

Lemon balm: Used for treating anxiety, insomnia, and digestive problems.

Nettle: Used for treating allergies, arthritis, and inflammation.

Peppermint: Used for treating digestive problems, headaches, and nausea.

Rosemary: Used for treating headaches, indigestion, and joint pain.

Thyme: Used for treating cough, sore throat, and respiratory infections.

Turmeric: Used for treating inflammation and digestive problems.

Valerian: Used for treating anxiety, insomnia, and nervous system disorders.

Witch hazel: Used for treating skin irritations, insect bites, and bruises.

Yellow dock: Used for treating skin conditions and digestive problems.

Willow bark: Used for treating pain, fever, and inflammation.

Echinacea: Used to boost the immune system and alleviate cold and flu symptoms.

Yarrow: Used to stop bleeding and promote wound healing.

Plantain: Used as an anti-inflammatory to relieve insect bites, stings, and rashes.

Arnica: Used to reduce pain and inflammation associated with bruises, sprains, and sore muscles.

Goldenseal: Used as an antimicrobial and anti-inflammatory to treat infections and soothe sore throats.

Comfrey: Used to promote healing of cuts, bruises, and sprains.

St. John's Wort: Used as an antidepressant and to relieve nerve pain.

Chamomile: Used as a relaxant and to relieve anxiety, insomnia, and stomach upset.

Licorice: Used to soothe sore throats and digestive issues.

Eucalyptus: Used as an expectorant to relieve congestion and cough.

Sage: Used to soothe sore throats, reduce sweating, and improve digestion.

Lavender: Used as a relaxant, to relieve headaches and insomnia, and to soothe skin irritation.

Catnip: Used as a relaxant and to soothe stomach upset.

Mullein: Used as an expectorant to relieve coughs and congestion.

Black cohosh: Used to relieve menstrual cramps and menopausal symptoms.

Milk thistle: Used to support liver function and to detoxify the body.

Red clover: Used to support overall health and as a blood thinner.

Devil's claw: Used as an anti-inflammatory to relieve joint pain and muscle aches.

Marshmallow root: Used to soothe sore throats and digestive issues.

Passionflower: Used as a relaxant to relieve anxiety and insomnia.

Saw palmetto: Used to support prostate health and to relieve urinary tract symptoms.

Dandelion root: Used as a diuretic to support kidney function and to detoxify the body.

Horehound: Used as an expectorant to relieve coughs and congestion.

It is important to remember that the use of alternative medications via plants requires extra study and investigation around their effectiveness. Please always consult with a medical expert when it comes to making important decisions about your health and safety.

About the Author

Antonio is a father of two children who he loves dearly. He has been working in the field of education for almost twenty-five years, primarily with students ages K-21. He believes that basic first aid education is the key to saving more lives all over the world. The simple act of knowing what to do in an emergency situation could be all the difference for the life of someone you love very dearly. It is his hope that one day, every hospital and school will hand out this handbook to every patient or student, just so they have the basics to support, or possibly save, the life of another. Education is truly the most powerful tool we have to transform the future.

Disclaimer

Please note that the advice provided is intended for informational purposes only and should not be taken as legal or professional advice. It is important to always seek the guidance of a qualified professional when making decisions that may have legal consequences. Additionally, it is important to use your own judgment and intuition when making any decisions, as ultimately you are responsible for the outcome. Please consult with a qualified professional before making any decisions that may have legal or other significant consequences. This disclaimer is not intended to limit or exclude any liability that may not be excluded or limited by law.

This handbook was a collaboration between the author and an open AI platform, with the sole purpose of trying to save more lives, by educating everyone who picks up this handbook on how to act in an emergency situation if ever called upon.

First Edition: 2023
ISBN: 9798374371468

Content Feedback: Please direct all feedback to www.handbooksforhumanity.com

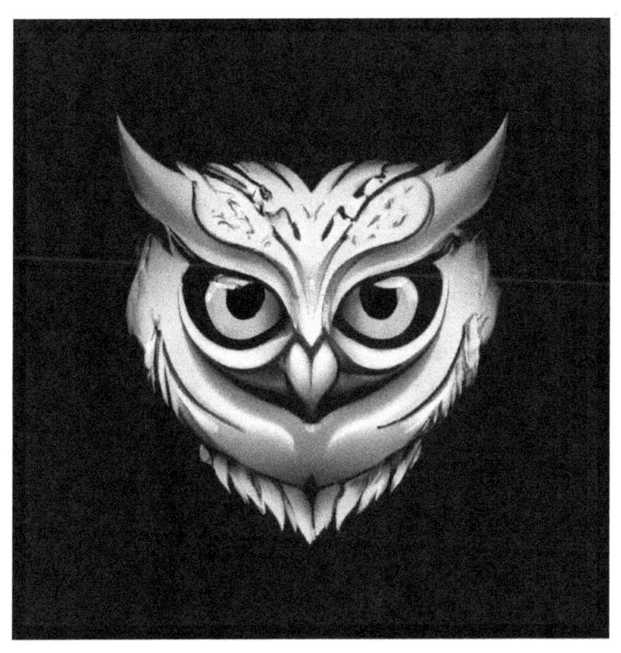

Copyright © 2023

Gufo Publishing

www.ingramcontent.com/pod-product-compliance
Lightning Source LLC
Chambersburg PA
CBHW050813250726
48653CB00006B/2204